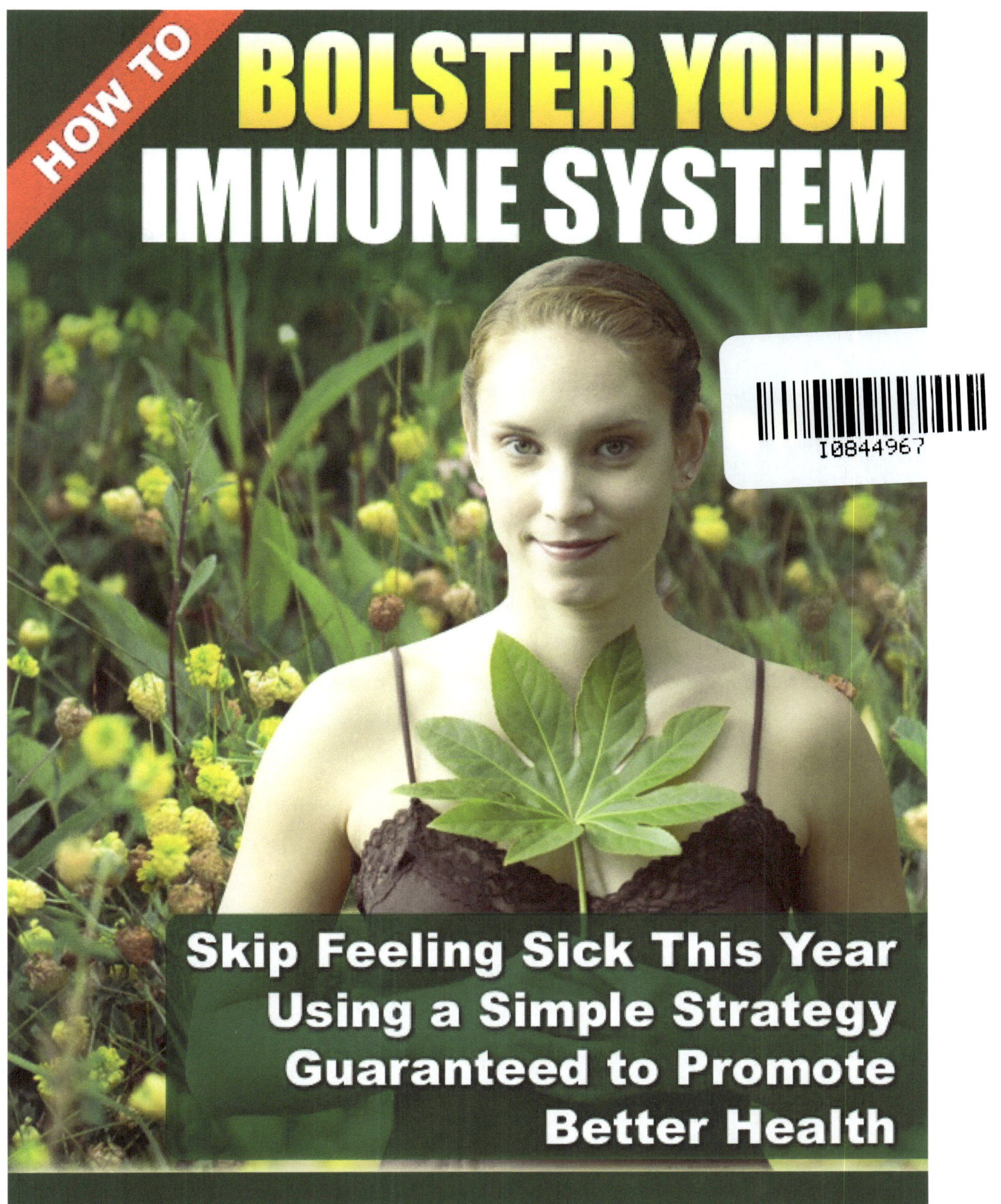

HOW TO
BOLSTER YOUR
IMMUNE SYSTEM
I0844967
Skip Feeling Sick This Year
Using a Simple Strategy
Guaranteed to Promote
Better Health
By : Franki Robert

## *Terms and Conditions*

The information contained in this guide is for information purposes only, and may not apply to your situation. The author, publisher, distributor and provider provide no warranty about the content or accuracy of content enclosed. Information contained herein is subjective. Keep this in mind when reviewing this guide.

The information in this guide is not provided as medical advice. You should always consult with your doctor if you have a health condition that requires treatment. The authors, publishers and owners of this guide are not medical doctors, psychologists or psychotherapists of any kind, and are not qualified to provide medical, psychological or therapeutic advice. You agree to hold all parties associated with creation and sales of this guide free from liability associated with any physical, mental, emotional, psychological or other harm arising from use of this guide or the website.

Neither the Publisher nor Author shall be liable for any loss of profit or any other commercial damages resulting from use of this guide.  All links are for information purposes only. We do not warrant for content, accuracy or any other implied or explicit purpose.

# Table of Contents

# Introduction

*"While we may not be able to control all that happens to us, we can control what happens inside us…" – Benjamin Franklin*

As Benjamin Franklin suggests, while it is impossible at times to control the many things that happen, we do have some control over what happens inside our bodies. Our bodies are a reflection of our inner health. If we eat well and exercise, our bodies are more likely to perform well.

When we eat junk food and forget to care for our bodies, fail to wash our hands or engage in other activities that promote sickness, often we become sick. Most people give up during the winter, with the feeling that it is impossible to stay healthy and not get sick. This simply isn't true.

## Your Body May Always Be Under Attack… But You CAN Fight Back…

No matter the time of year your body is always susceptible to attack; it could be the common cold, the flu, food poisoning or some other virus you contracted at the play ground while watching your best friend's four year old. Disease is everywhere. That doesn't mean you are powerless to control disease. There are many steps you can take to bolster your immune system yearly. What are these steps?

We'll talk more about them later. First, you have to understand how disease works and when you are most likely to become ill. Once you understand this everything else will fall into place. So, when are you most susceptible to illness?

During winter people are more likely to become symptomatic largely because they are indoors. Without adequate ventilation, anybody that stays indoors for any length of time is subject to attack. Some people are also sedentary more so in the winter than at other times during the year when the weather is warm and inviting. If you find you are a couch potato during the cold, winter months, you are probably more at risk for illness. Unless you follow proper hygiene habits and ventilate your home daily.

Even if you do this, there are no guarantees you will not get sick. If however, your body is in good shape, you may be able to reduce the severity of your illness.

Anyone can become sick any time of the year however, even during the warm months of summer. While it sound's scary, there is good news. Our body's immune systems are always ready to attack foreign invaders. Unless your immune system is compromised (as is often the case with patients that have autoimmune disorders) the chances are not high you will have to fight the virus you contracted at your office party for months on end.

Most people, even those that do not use medication, will overcome the common cold and similar viruses within a week to ten days.

If you do have a disease that comoromises your immune system you are more at risk for disease, but this does not mean you have to succumb to disease. You can still fight back, and you should fight back. The methods you employ to foster good health however, may be more stringent than those offered in this guide alone. Be sure to talk to your healthcare specialist if you suffer from a disease that makes it difficult for your immune system to fight the common cold and other foreign invaders.

There are of course many other organisms besides viruses that can attack your body, including bacteria. Fortunately bacterial infections are typically treatable with antibiotics. While medication only alleviates symptoms in most viral attacks, medication usually wipes out bacteria or the cause of attacks in patients with these types of disorders.

### The Problem with Antibiotics

Antibiotics are sometimes considered a "panacea," which means people think they are a form of medicine capable of killing all forms of disease. This is not true.

While there are many antibiotics available to treat disease, they are effective for killing diseases resulting from bacteria, not those forming from viruses.

There is no antibiotic that helps cure a viral infection. If you take an antibiotic when you have a viral cold, you may build up antibodies so that when your body does fall ill because of a bacterial infection, the antibiotic your doctor normally might use may not work.

Bacteria are organisms that grow, change and mature. They are especially good at adaptation. That means they can adapt to their surroundings, becoming more powerful. When this happens many antibiotics that used to be able to cure an infection are no longer able to. Today there are only a handful of antibiotics available to treat some of the more dangerous diseases.

This is largely due to overuse of antibiotics. Many doctors feel pressured to prescribe them to patients that demand an antibiotic to feel better. The patient does not sometimes realize the antibiotic may have a placebo effect, meaning they feel better even though there recovery has nothing to do with the antibiotic.

Alternatively, the person may feel better because by the time they take the antibiotic, there body may already be successfully fighting the virus that first invaded the body.

Antibiotics are not something to fool around with. If you can find a suitable solution to your ailment without using them, then use it, with your doctor's approval.

Now that you understand how important it is to prevent illness and prepare your body to fight illness, let's see how you would go about doing just that.

### Can You Bolster Your Immune System?

It **IS** possible to strengthen your body so you are less likely to develop a cold, or at least if you do your body will return to health faster than the "average" bear. This guide is a tool anyone can use to help fight back against the common cold, flu, bacterial diseases, food born illness or poisoning and more. Please note before we continue, if you are sick you should always check in with your doctor or other medical healthcare provider.

Your doctor or healthcare authority is the person in charge of your health. We've done our best to provide you with helpful and relevant information in this guide; however the author and publisher of this guide are not doctors. Remember that. If you are taking any kind of medication or being treated for a specific illness or chronic disease, make sure you talk to your doctor about any of the tips provided before you start using them.

Got it? Good. This book is a compilation of years worth of research into the human body and the connection between mind, body and spirit. No, we aren't talking religion in case you were wondering. What we mean is simple: by identifying the causes for illness rather than just treating the symptoms, you bolster your mind, you physical body and your spirit, otherwise known as your gut or your subconscious.

All human body systems work in harmony with each other, usually to help protect you from disease. While we can't infuse aromatherapy oils or vitamin C into the air filters at your job, we can provide you with some solid information about tools people have used successfully to bolster their immune systems. Keep in mind every person is unique, so what works for one person may not work as well for another person. You must find out what methods or tools work best for you and your body.

## Always seek medical advice before attempting to treat or cure an illness…

Remember that your doctor is the one person that is most qualified to diagnose an illness. Your doctor can tell you if he or she suspects a viral or bacterial infection.

Now it is time to review the various tools available to you; these are tools anyone can use to help bolster their immune system. The tools and practices in this guide do not come with a guarantee. They may not work for everyone. But, most people find these tools and techniques are beneficial and helpful for preventing disease or shortening the length of a disease that already exists (like the common cold, which really isn't that common).

Are you ready to take a peak?

Before you begin go grab a highlighter. You may find parts of this book more helpful to you than others, so be sure to make a point to highlight them. You can at the very least create your own "to do" or "to check into" list if you read about

immune boosting strategies you think will help you while you attempt to conquer
your illness.

# Chapter 1 – Understanding Our Immune System

Before you learn how you can defend your immune system from foreign invaders, you must first understand how your immune system works. When you do this you can use several tools, including visualization and meditation techniques to improve your body's health and ability to fight disease, no matter its origin.

Our immune systems are central to our livelihood. When we care for them properly, they do exactly as we want them to. Even if we fall ill, when we are healthy most of the time, our bodies respond by fighting diseases and bacterial agents much harder. Since most people probably haven't taken a biology or anatomy class for some time, let's stop for a moment to find out how the immune system works.

It is really quite easy, easier than most people think.

## *Your Internal Bio-Powered Immune Fighting Machine*

If we took perfect care of our bodies we would soon realize our bodies are bio-powered immune fighting machines, stronger than any antioxidant or antibiotic out there. We are made to instinctively gather food, care for our loved ones and offspring, and combat or fight against any invaders, whether visible or invisible to the human eye.

### Our bodies were built to fight off infection and disease.

How do our bodies do this? It's easy.

Let's find out how your body works to find any type of bacterial or viral agent that may enter.

Bacterial and viral agents can enter the body many different ways. Don't think you are safe just because you wash your hands a few times a day.

Look at the following example which illustrates in a few simple steps what happens when disease enters your body.

1) Bacteria or viral organisms enter your body through touch, sneezes, physical contact or through other mechanisms. Keep in mind if someone coughs, their phlegm may spread 500 feet, meaning whatever illness they have will shower the people around them unless they cover their mouths. That is why it is so important to close your mouth and cover your mouth if you have to cough or sneeze.

2) Your body's immune system receives a signal from your brain that shouts out "Time to make white blood cells!" White blood cells are the types of cells in your body that react to infection. Their job is to help create cells that fight diseases whether they are viral or bacterial in nature.

3) Your body also starts producing antibodies, which are specific types of white blood cells that fight off infection. Antibodies, including IgE help fight allergies and other disorders. IgA is a type of antibody that commonly helps fight against infection.

4) If your immune system is as strong as it can be, your body will send enough antibodies and white blood cells to fight any attack, no matter how severe. This doesn't mean you won't get sick, it means your body will do everything it can to keep you healthy. If you get sick, the chances are high you will recover much faster if your immune system is working wonders.

5) It may take you a few days to recover, but most people recover from minor infections or viruses relatively easily. It may take from 7 to 10 days for the average cold or bacterial infection. Immuno-compromised patients may find it takes their body much longer to overcome something as simple as the common cold.

Now, most people do not have a fine-tuned immune system. If you had one you probably wouldn't need to read this guide, now would you? This guide will help you "fine tune" your immune system so you have the best chances of reducing the length of an illness or preventing an illness all at the same time. Now that you understand how the immune system works, you should learn about the many factors that influence your immune system. These are elements that may make your immune system function less optimally than you would like.

### *Factors That Influence Your Immune System*

Your immune system may be compromised in many ways. Here are some reasons your body may not jump to attack an infection or disease they way you think it should.

Remember, you may engage in only one or two of these habits, but they will still impact your immune system negatively. Some people will fall ill even if their immune systems are attacked minimally, a result of one or two poor habits. Here are some examples.

> ➢ **You eat too much fast food or incorporate too much saturated fat into your diet**. Fat can clog your arteries, contribute to type II diabetes and increase the total body fat you carry around with you.

- ➢ **You rarely exercise, and when you do you do so half-heartedly, or you over do it, which can cause you to become ill rather than prevent illness**. Sometimes more is better; however, more is not better if you exercise to the point where you over train your muscles and body. You need to give your body a break, especially between strength training sessions, so you are able to fight against disease.

- ➢ **You thrive on stress, which sends levels of cortisol (a stress hormone) through the roof, which can result in general malaise or illness**. Stress is a killer. In fact, stress can lead to heart attacks, high blood pressure, anger and aggression, depression and many other disorders. The less stressed you are the better your body will be at fighting disease.

- ➢ **You don't sleep enough, which also changes the hormone levels in your body.** This inspires you to eat more and increases your susceptibility to common colds or infections. You may gain weight, which also puts you at risk for diseases like type II diabetes.

- ➢ **You sleep too much, which doesn't allow your body the physical activity it needs to get going and perform at its best.** It IS important to sleep. However, if you find you sleep more than 10 hours each day, you may have a health problem. You should consult with your doctor. Most people do well when they sleep 6-8 hours each day, preferably closer to the 7 to 8 range.

- ➢ **You don't eat enough or you eat too much, so your body doesn't receive the fuel it needs to fight disease.** The good news is you don't have to deprive yourself of all the luxuriant foods in life to be healthy; you just have to use a practical approach, one that encourages moderation in all things. When you deprive yourself of food for too long, your body goes into starvation mode. This actually slows DOWN your metabolism, meaning you will gain weight even if you eat less portions than you have in the past.

It sounds a bit technical, but when you look at your immune system as a complex machine, which it is, you are more likely to take care of and fine tune it. You would put oil in your car if it needed it, wouldn't you? The same premise applies here. You have to care for your body just as you would any other appliance or other object that belongs to you (that you care about).

If you don't care for your body and perform maintenance checks (annual physicals) you are more likely to develop illnesses that you might have been able to prevent. Your doctor may find something comes up in your blood tests that you may not have known had you not visited the doctor to begin with. You can skimp on many things in life. You can skimp on extra cheese; you can try spending a little less money. One thing you must invest in however, is your health. When your health is good, you feel good. When you feel good, you can do almost anything your heart desires.

Now it's time to learn the steps you have to take to ensure your wellness. If you follow the steps provided in the next chapter, you will be well on your way to a happy, healthy and bountiful future. Are you ready to take on the challenge? Then keep reading (I hope you said yes) to find out what you need to do to take on the world with health and with vigor.

# Chapter 3 – Step-by-Step Health Regimen

Your immune system is your best friend when you want to help protect your body against colds, influenza and other common illnesses that often strike young children, the elderly and people with compromised immune systems. Keep in mind, if you don't eat well and exercise, you might as well consider yourself compromised.

Don't worry about labeling yourself; that isn't important. It is more important you understand the steps you have to take to lead a healthier and cleaner life. Here is how you do that.

## *Step 1: Wash Your Hands*

It's no joke. The first step is the easiest step to follow, and you may feel like rolling your eyes.

However, the #1 way people get sick is by hand-to-hand contact. You may shake the hand of someone that is ill and forget to wash your hands before you eat your midday snack.

You may hold your child's hand while going to the park, play on the equipment (which may contain several hundred different kinds of viruses or bacteria) and then sit down for a picnic without washing your hands.

These are bad habits, very bad habits. These are the kind of habits that will cause you to become ill. You and every member of your family should always wash your hands, especially if someone in the house is sick. Here are some times where it is critical for you to wash your hands.

- **Any time you go out of doors and return home**. This is especially true if you go to crowded places.

- **Any time you and/or your children go to the park**. If you want to have a picnic and there is nowhere handy to wash hands, then pass around some moist towlettes. You can find these almost anywhere. These are great for use when on-the-go. Another new invention is miniature bottles of sanitizer. You can buy pocket sized sanitizer and give one to each member of the family. You just squirt a tiny bit in your palms and rub them clean, no water or rinsing required. Some even come with built in lotion or aloe to promote softness for your hands during cold winter months.

- **When you go out to eat**. Any time you decide to go out to eat you should wash your hands before you eat your food. Again, this is an environment where you can easily use a moist towel or take a trip to the restroom to clean up before you eat.

- **When caring for a loved one that is ill**. Sometimes while caring for the people we love most, we forget how important it is to care for ourselves. However, you can spread illness by caring for someone and then touching another person if you do not wash your hands.

- **When handling pets or pet material**. Pets are lovely to have, but they often harbor many diseases. Make sure you wash your hands after touching the family dog.

- **Before planning and preparing meals**. You should always wash your hands before and after handling food products you plan to eat or to serve others. If you are ill you may contaminate everyone else in the household. Be especially careful when preparing foods that have a meat and a vegetable part. Raw meat may harbor many diseases including salmonella or E. coli to name a few. Make sure you do not use the same cutting board when preparing vegetables compared with meats. Each should have its own special cutting board.

### Step 2 – Eat Immune Boosting Foods

There are many immune boosting foods anyone can eat. These foods will not cure a cold immediately, but they may prepare your body to fight harder against diseases.

Most people know that fruits, whole grains and vegetables top the list of must eat items. Some people believe that chicken soup makes you well when you are sick.

Other people still live by the old adage "starve a cold and feed a fever." So what should you eat? Here is a list of the foods that are most likely to result in better health. These foods have proven beneficial for bolstering one's overall wellness, which in turn may help boost the odds you will be able to fight infection or viruses if they attack.

- **Fish or Flax** – these foods provide essential fatty acids, which are tiny substances that are wonderful for reducing inflammation in the body, a common cause for illness. While you can take a supplement containing Omega-3 fatty acids (a key essential fatty acid) you can also get essential fatty acids from your diet. Some good sources of fatty acids in food include fatty fishes like tuna, salmon and mackerel.

- **Yogurt** – yogurt contains ingredients called probiotics that help balance the flora in the digestive tract. When the flora in the body becomes uncontrolled, diseases like yeast infections or UTI become common.

- **Mushrooms** – Eastern medical practitioners often use Shitake mushrooms to bolster the immune system. Most mushrooms contain vitamin B and many other essential nutrients. You will benefit whether you eat the Shitake variety or any other variety, as long as you incorporate them into an overall healthy diet.

- **Fresh fruits** – especially blueberries, strawberries and bananas, all of which contain powerful ingredients to bolster the immune system and help the body fight back against disease. Blueberries, raspberries and strawberries contain many antioxidants; theses are substances that reduce free radical damage. Free radical damage is damage that occurs on the surface of an object. Free radical damage can occur from too much unprotected exposure to the sun or other environmental pollutants. Bananas contain plenty of potassium, which helps balance the electrolytes in your body.

- **Seaweed** – some believe seaweed (often used in Eastern dishes like sushi) contains ingredients that bolster the action of T cells in the body; these are disease fighting cells. Seaweed may also cause the body to produce more antibodies, which are a type of white blood cell that helps fight disease and infection.

- **Herbs** – herbs are powerful substances anyone can use to flavor dishes and combat disease. There are certain herbs like cumin, cayenne and cilantro that may help bolster circulation and improve one's immunity. This is especially true of cayenne, which heats the body. Some believe cayenne may help increase the metabolism also, which is why it is an ingredient in many natural health supplements promoting weight loss benefits.

- **Green Tea** – this tea, like many other teas, is a powerhouse of antioxidants. Black tea also contains many beneficial antioxidants, but studies suggest green tea is best. You can buy it decaf or caffeinated. Green tea is often used in weight loss products because many believe it stimulates the metabolic system. The antioxidants in the tea may help ward off infection or illness. Sipping tea with a bit of honey and lemon while sick can soothe an itchy, red or sore throat.

- **Water** – it may sound crazy, but many people mistake thirst for hunger and overeat. Water, pure, filtered and clean water is one of the best substances you can drink if you want to stay well or get better faster. Water hydrates the body. Most people, especially those living in dry climates, do not drink enough water. Water is essential for every biological process that occurs in the body. Water helps the digestive system work properly.

  It helps your skin feel healthy and it helps your body recover from illness. If you don't like the taste of water there are many products now promoting water with added flavors you can try. Just be sure you don't indulge in one that has a lot of calories, or you will pack on pounds. If you are dehydrated however, some people find an electrolyte enhanced drink like Gatorade or similar products help replenish the system. You can even drink some water with a pinch of sea salt and lemon to help balance the electrolytes in your body.

- **Garlic and Onion** – fresh garlic has many immune boosting properties, whether you take it as a supplement or as a whole food. If you get fresh garlic and fry it or add it to favorite foods including sauces, you will give your immune system a power boost. Garlic has antifungal, antibacterial and energy boosting qualities. When combined with onion in light broth, many people find it helps relieve sinus congestion or lessens the amount of time they suffer from a cold. When in doubt, always go for the garlic, and take a breath freshener with you while out and about.

- **Oats and Barley** – These are whole grains containing loads of a healthy fiber that contains antioxidants and antimicrobial ingredients. Many feel oats and barley are more beneficial then Echinacea. Some studies suggest oats and barley may be helpful with people with compromised immune systems, or those that are susceptible to the flue and similar illnesses.

This list is far from comprehensive, but it does give you an idea of the types of foods you can eat that are most likely to result in better health. You should think about eating whole foods rather than processed or packaged foods, as many processed foods (even if fortified with vitamins) contain too much fat and too many preservatives.

Whole foods include foods that are in their whole state; they are natural, minimally processed and good for you. You can find grains, vegetables and lean proteins that are whole foods. Look for meat that does not contain much in the way of antibiotics. Many meats processed by traditional stores are laden with hormones to help the cows providing the meat and milk to grow.

These hormones do not disappear; so, if you feed your child whole milk that has been pasteurized and comes from a cow that feeds on antibiotics or growth hormones, your child may ingest the same hormones. Some researchers believe this is one reason why so many young adolescents are hitting puberty much earlier in life.

## Organic vs. Non-Organic

If you've been to any grocer in the last year or more you've probably noticed some changes. One change that is welcomed by many is the introduction of organic foods as an alternative to traditional foods.

You can now purchase organically grown fruits, vegetables, dairy products and some proteins or meats. What is the difference?

Most organic foods are grown on organic farms. These farms do not use heavy chemicals or pesticides to prevent insects from affecting the plant. They are grown without the addition of hormones to improve the size or shape of the product.

That means your cucumber may be a bit smaller than normal and your tomato may look a little uneven or asymmetrical; however, organic foods are allowed to grow to their full potential before offered to the public. You do not have to worry about ingesting or feeding your family food that is contaminated with unwanted pollutants.

People are becoming more conscious of organic foods. Many feel they simply taste better than conventional foods, and they do. They are however, a bit pricier than non-organic alternatives. If you find you have a limited budget, you can sample organic foods by first trying some organic meats and/or dairy products. These are the foods most likely to contain hormones you probably prefer you and your child not eat.

If you buy as part of a co-op, where several people pay a smaller amount of money to receive a box of various vegetables and fruits, you can save money buying these items. Ask around your neighborhood or visit a local farmers market to find out if any organization like this exists in your home town.

You can also learn more about co-op's online. Here are some sites to visit and learn more about this process. All of the sites below provide tools you can use to locate organic farmers or co-op nurseries in your area if you live in the United States. Some even offer information about organic production and distribution abroad.

- www.coopdirectory.org
- www.localharvest.org
- www.organicconsumers.org/purelink.html

You can even have organic foods prepared and delivered right to your door. Many organizations deliver boxed goods containing a wide variety of organic products.

You can also order pre-cooked meals online. Here is an example of a site that does just that:

www.theorganicdish.com

It's almost like any other prepared food service, like weight watchers, however with this program you get organic ingredients and meals delivered right to your door. You may also look in your local phone book, as many organizations like this are sprouting in small and large cities that have an inclination toward natural and organic foods and lifestyles.

## Step 3 – Take Your Vitamins & Supplements

Eating well is critical to your health; so is taking the right vitamins and supplements. During various stages of our life we all need a little extra pizzazz. You should always talk with your healthcare provider before you use any over-the-counter supplement.

This is especially true if you take prescription medications regularly, because some supplements or vitamins may negatively interact with each other. Some supplements may reduce or increase the side effects of prescription medications, as can some foods. So be sure you talk to your doctor before you try any of these.

A qualified healthcare provider can also guide you by telling you how much of a vitamin or supplement you need to take to realize better help or to bolster your immune system.

Below is a list of some of the more common supplements recommended to people for boosting the immune system.

- **Probiotics** – Sometimes referred to as "acidophilus" or other related substances, probiotics help balance the natural flora or good bacteria that resides in the body. Often when someone takes antibiotics, the antibiotic kills off all bacteria in the body, both good and bad. Unfortunately, good bacteria are needed for proper digestion and elimination. Some studies suggest the use of probiotics in children and in adults may reduce digestive disease risk, improve immunity to common ailments and may even reduce the number of infectious diseases that cause fever in people that take them regularly[i].

- **Omega-3 fatty acid** – a supplement containing omega-3 like fish oil or flax seed oil can improve your overall health and wellness. Essential fatty acids like this also help reduce inflammation in the body. Often doctors recommend patients with arthritis or related illnesses take an anti-inflammatory agent like essential fatty acids.

- **Vitamin C** – vitamin C is one of the cheapest and easiest ways to get your daily serving of immune boosting ingredients. There is much controversy in the health community about how much vitamin C is enough vitamin C to protect the body. One way to gauge this is to take one tablet a day ,and increase your dose until you feel abdominal discomfort. However, this may not work for all people. It is best you speak with your healthcare professional about the proper dose of vitamin C for you based on your health and body weight.

- **Echinacea** – this herb has been promoted as a virtual panacea for all ailments. If taken regularly during a cold it may help reduce the length or severity of a cold. You can buy it as an herb or in capsule and tincture formulations. Most healthcare providers recommend you do not take this year 'round, because it may lose its ability to fight disease if taken daily. If you are ill, you might consider taking it for a week and then taking a week off to see how well you do. Studies about Echinacea are controversial; some people swear by its effectiveness and others doubt it helps at all. Keep in mind all bodies are different. If you take it and it seems to help, then use it. If you find it doesn't then try something else.

- **Goldenseal** – this is a powerful herb that you should use with caution. Manufacturers note it has antibacterial and antiseptic properties. It can cause digestive upset, and should not be taken during pregnancy as it can promote contractions or early labor. Goldenseal is a species that is dying out, so it is important to take it when needed, and to only take as much as you need to feel well. A trained herbalist can work with you to find out what the best dose is for your body type.

- **Zinc** – many people have zinc deficiencies which may cause fatigue and lethargy. Many cold formulas at stores now offer zinc as a primary ingredient. This is true of many tablets used to soothe a sore throat. It is sometimes difficult to get enough zinc from the food you eat, so if you are sick you may find it helps to take a little extra zinc. Often you can find a zinc lozenge.

If you want to learn more about supplements and herbs that may help bolster your immune system you should consider finding a qualified natural healthcare provider or consult with an herbalist before you buy anything.

You will find there are many other supplements on the market that claim they boost health and wellness. Some of these contain a mixture of ingredients or herbs and natural vitamins and minerals. Before you buy a supplement after hours of searching the shelves of a health food store, talk to a qualified herbalist or other health care practitioner. He or she can help you decide what, if any, supplement will help you best as you try to overcome your illness. Only someone that is qualified and understands basic anatomy and physiology, and the drug interactions likely to occur when someone takes an herb with a medication, can really assist you as you try to find the best immunity formula to suit your needs.

You can also ask what herbs you can use or foods you can use to help prevent disease (like shitake mushrooms and seaweed). Some foods and supplements (including garlic) are sometimes better taken as a preventive medicine than as a cure for any illness.

Speaking of garlic, you may also consider adding more garlic to your diet, whether in the form of a capsule or raw garlic. Garlic acts in much the same way that goldenseal does; many consider it natures natural antibiotic. Just be careful not to eat too much at once because it may upset your stomach.

Many newer supplements containing garlic are now odorless and tasteless, so you don't have to worry about scaring off the vampires with your garlic perfume, if you will.

Now that you have an idea of what types of supplements you can take to improve your immunity, let's look at the next two steps you can take to help your immune system punch out disease. Are you ready?

## *Step 4 – Exercise*

You knew it would come at some point or another, the great lecture on exercise. First, do not think of this as a lecture. This book is a tool you can use to help improve your health and wellness. It is not something that you should dread. Everyone needs to exercise.

We will not tell you how well you are exercising or what type of exercising is best for you. You are better off asking your doctor that question. We can however, let you in on a little secret – a little exercise will boost your immune system. That's true whether you exercise one hour a day or 10 minutes 7 days each week.

Even if you are skinny, you may need to get more exercise. Many people assume that because they are skinny they should not have to exercise much to stay in shape. Quite the opposite is true however. There are many "skinny" people walking around that are "fat" on the inside, and the inside is what counts. You can have a high body fat percentage and still "look" skinny. Why is this? Muscle weighs more than fat.

Someone that is 120 pounds and 14% lean looks very different from someone that is 120 pounds and has 30 % body fat. The person with 30 percent body fat may be just under five feet tall, but based on the body fat calculation they are obese.

If you want a true measure of how healthy you are (which predicts your odds of staying in great shape and fighting disease) you should ask your doctor to offer you a body fat measurement and a BMI calculation.

Once you find out what these numbers are, you can start a reasonable exercise program; say 20 minutes of exercise 3 days each week. Eventually you will find exercise enjoyable and can work your way up the ladder, working out 30 minutes instead of 20 minutes. The cycle continues.

BMI stands for body mass index. It is a tool many doctors and therapists use to assess how fit or unfit a person's body is. There are many free calculators you can use on the web to calculate your body mass index, including ones from the Centers for Disease Control, American Heart Association, and National Institutes of Health.

Here are a couple of links you can follow to learn more:

- **CDC Adult & Child BMI Calculators**
  www.cdc.gov/nccdphp/dnpa/bmi - this is a great site with loads of free information on calculating BMI and fat mass for children and adults. You can also learn more about the many different diseases there are that are susceptible to weight changes. You might also learn more about infectious diseases and how to prevent them.

- **Adult BMI Calculator UK**
  www.health.nsw.gov.au/obesity/adult/bmi.html

As with any calculator this allows you to calculate your BMI in kilograms or in pounds if you convert the figures. This site also offers information on childhood obesity and tips for overcoming obesity and overweight.

**➡ Youth BMI Calculator UK**

www.health.nsw.gov.au/obesity/youth/bmi.html

This is a great tool for parents interested in finding out how healthy their child is. You can use the tool on this page to calculate the BMI for children and young adults to age 18. It is important to note calculations for young children are different from those adults use.

The National Institute of Health also provides a written explanation of how to calculate your body mass index manually. While most people prefer the ol' calculator, may doctors or healthcare providers will calculate BMI manually or by using a special "map" of the human body that outlines or separates healthy weights from unhealthy weights. If you want to find out what your BMI is manually just follow the formula below.

1. First, weigh yourself, write that number down.
2. Next, multiply your weight in pounds by the number 703.
3. Now, divide the answer you get by your height (calculated in inches).
4. Finally, divide the answer from step 3 by your height again (in inches).

This is a long but not difficult process. If you want quick information you may find the BMI online calculators much faster.

You can measure your body fat with calipers, which most doctors and physical trainers have. There are other ways of calculating body fat, but most are long and cumbersome. Most doctors or physical therapists offer body fat testing if you ask them. If they do not, find someone that does or ask your doctor for a referral. You can buy your own caliper online, but if you do keep in mind you may have trouble distinguishing fat from muscle mass or skin.

That means you are more likely to get an inaccurate reading if you measure your body fat alone, unless you are already a health professional well-versed in body fat calculations. The BMI with the body fat analysis is the best predictor of health for most people. The BMI is often not the best choice for athletes because they may weigh a lot and still look skinny, resulting from the higher than average muscle mass in their bodies.

## What Exercises Boost the Immune System?

So far we've touched on everything EXCEPT the exercises you can engage in to boost your immune system. There are many exercises anyone can participate in and have a good time with.

The type of exercise you select will depend on many things including your current health, your medical history and your physical activity history. If you've never exercised a day in your life, your best bet may be walking. While this seems controversial it is not. The more people walk, the more likely they are to be healthy. When we say "walk" we do not mean stroll or casually glide along the walkway.

When you walk for exercise you should walk as fast as you can, almost to the point where you are jogging, so you get your heart rate up, provided this is safe for you. You can pump your arms to increase the effects your walking has on your health.

You should ask your physician or other healthcare provider for some advice when power walking so you know how long to walk and whether you can enjoy other exercises besides walking. Here is a list of exercises people commonly enjoy. These will help keep you in shape which naturally will help improve your ability to fight off infection.

1. **Swimming** – light swimming is great because it is easy on the joints and works every muscle group. If you are not able to swim you can still get in the pool and enjoy an aqua aerobics or related class to help you get in the swing of things.

2. **Stair Climbing** – provided you have strong knees you can climb outdoors where the air is fresh. If you have a school with a football stadium near you climb up and down the stairs on a nice day.

3. **Walking or Jogging** – many people find they start walking and eventually end jogging. Jogging on a grassy surface or other soft terrain (sand or soil) is easier on the knees than walking on pavement.

4. **Biking** – you can bike indoors or out. Try a reclined bike which allows you to sit in a way that doesn't harm your body. This type of cycle allows you to sit at an angle instead of straight up and down, so it is much easier to stay on the bike for long sessions.

5. **Strength Training** – this is an important part of any exercise program especially if you want to lose fat and improve your muscle mass. You can start out using machines and graduate to free weights. Make sure you have someone show you how to do an exercise correctly before you try doing something yourself. You may end up sorry if you do not. Strength training can be fun and exciting, but not if you tear a muscle.

6. **Yoga** – yoga is a wonderful form of exercise that can improve your immunity and help improve your body's flexibility. Many of the poses are

cleansing and gentle, ideal for someone that would like a moving meditation.

7. **Pilates** – like yoga, this is a powerful exercise that can boost the body's immune system and lengthen muscles. You can work to correct muscle imbalances and realize greater strength.

8. **Tai Chi** – this is a meditative practice much like yoga but is much gentler, allowing the person participating to enjoy a standing meditation while also moving in gentle postures and flow. Tai Chi purportedly can help restore the natural alignment of energies in the body.

9. **Meditation** – many people do not consider meditation exercise. That is because they are looking at meditation the wrong way. Meditation is exercise; it is exercise for the body, mind and soul. When we allow ourselves to meditate, we feed our minds and provide our body with an opportunity to rest, relax and rejuvenate. We also decrease stress, which is necessary if you want to improve your immunity to common ailments.

10. **Visualization** – exercises for the mind include visualization exercises. You can imagine your body fighting back against disease. Just close your eyes, create an image of your perfect, healthy body, and hold that vision close to your mind and heart. The mind is very powerful. When we believe using our minds that we are well and free of disease, most times our bodies respond accordingly.

Your body, mind and spirit need daily exercise to survive. If you focus on disease then you are more susceptible to disease. What you should be doing is focusing on health and conquering disease. Cancer patients are often taught visualization skills that help them overcome their disease. Cancer is a disease where certain cancer cells in the body, or abnormal cells grow out of control.

Gentle motions performed through Tai Chi, Yoga or a practice called Qigong (another type of Eastern exercise involving low-impact movement of energy) are sometimes more helpful for boosting immunity that vigorous exercise, which may actually increase the stress hormones circulating in your system. Gentle motion exercises as these are helpful for providing your body with more energy, which means you have more ability to fight off infection and feel your best. You can enjoy these exercises as much or as little as you want.

You can visualize disease or a chronic illness any way you want; the goal is to focus on getting rid of the cells responsible for your sickness or the virus and bacteria responsible for your lethargy. You can also perform visualizations where you imagine what your body would look like in a healthy state. You can imagine your perfect body, and then imagine you accomplishing any task you want with your perfect body. Many people with strong immune systems imagine their body is healthy whether it is or not.

Your subconscious can "trick" your brain into thinking you are healthy even if you are not healthy. It sounds strange, but it can happen. Doctors are using visualization techniques in hospitals to help patients recover faster. There are even studies suggesting visualization helps improve medical health and outcomes among patients with chronic illnesses.

**It is really a matter of mind over matter – in a literal way.**

Those opposing such techniques suggest visualization offers nothing more than a placebo would. The placebo effect is the feeling of something positive changing without anything actually changing. This can happen for many reasons. If people are given a medication and told it will cure their disease, they are more likely to realize positive health outcomes whether or not they receive medication or a sugar pill (at least in some cases).

The placebo effect does not happen for everyone, but it might work for you, even if you do not believe in visualizations to boost your immunity. What is the worst thing that can happen? You may end up right where you started, or you may find you feel a thousand times better.

## *Step 5 – Reduce Stress*

If you reduce the amount of stress you carry with you, you are more likely to feel better. Stress is a leading cause of illness in the United States and many others. It is important you realize how much stress impacts your life.

When you feel stressed, usually you have a harder than average time sleeping. If you can't sleep, then you can't function well during the day, and are more likely to become ill because your immune system is weak. With proper sleep and little stress however, your body is much more likely to respond positively and overcome any illness that may come its way.

How much stress do you carry around in your life?

**Stress Inventory –**

Find out what your stress triggers are, or how much stress you carry around with you daily, and you may improve the quality of your life and your health. Here are some common stress triggers. How many can you identify with?

1. Feeling tired or lethargic during the day even after a good night of sleep.

2. Worrying constantly about work assignments, school assignments or other activities that have a deadline.

3. Always arriving late to an event or meeting because you are scrambling to catch up on work that might have been done already had you not procrastinated.

4. You drink almost every night in excess to "relax" after a hard day's work.

5. Crying a lot for no reason, or feeling the blues constantly.

6. Falling behind your peers.

7. Feeling irritable or angrier than usual.

8. Driving recklessly or endangering yourself while driving or engaging in other ordinary activities.

9. Feeling like simple tasks are overly cumbersome.

10. Having trouble falling or staying asleep at night.

How many of these situations can you relate to? Stress is something you want to eliminate from your life as best you can. While you can't possibly rid the world of everything stressful, you can eliminate some of your stress, and some stress relief is better than no stress relief.

Here are some tips you can adopt to help release or reduce some of the stress in your life. The less stress you have the better your chance of fighting a cold.

Remember, none of these techniques guarantees you will not get sick; if you do get sick however, if you follow the advice offered in this guide you are more likely to recover much quicker than others.

- **Plan ahead**. If you have to go to work the next day, then pick out what you want to wear the night before, and make sure it is ironed and pressed so you are ready to go. That way you can sleep in or hit the snooze button at least once without running late.

- **Exercise daily.** You don't have to be a marathon runner to reap the benefits of exercise. All you really have to do is get outside for 15 minutes once or twice a day. Exercise helps bolster your body's immune system. When you exercise, you also feel better on the inside.

- **Organize and Prioritize**. If you have too much to do, you will find your tasks weigh you down. This can lead to stress, and stress contributes to illness. The most common argument people offer for not organizing is "I don't' have time". The reality is you do have time, especially if you want to get well. The less attention you pay to your body the more likely you are to stay sick. As long as you stay sick, you are going to suffer. If you take just 30 minutes out of each day to organize and prioritize, you will find your days flow much smoother. If you need help organizing, you can always ask a friend or family member to help out. Most will do so with gusto.

Naturally there are many other ways you can reduce stress. You can take a walk twice daily outside to get out of the house or your office building. You can take a 15 minute power nap. A power nap isn't really a nap. It is a small period of time you can use to recline, relax and kick back. The goal is not to think about the work ahead of you. Rather, you should spend the time focusing on creating more energy in your life. Imagine what your life would be like if you finished all of your tasks ahead of schedule. Once you do this, you are better able to manage the stress you do have on your plate without releasing too much in the way of cortisol or stress hormones.

Some people prefer traditional stress busters like a massage, pedicure or drive along the countryside. Any of these are a good idea. When you prepare for bed, try not to drink up to four hours before your head hits the pillow. While you may "think" the alcohol relaxes you, in the longer term it actually deprives you of much needed sleep. Alcohol only causes you to feel sleepy for a short time. Then it acts more like a stimulant, depriving you of deep sleep. You also develop a headache or become dehydrated, which can lead to even more stress.

You might consider setting up a bedtime ritual that involves meditation, a good read and silky sheets to relax in. Do whatever it is that appeals most to you to get the quality sleep you need. Speaking of sleep, let's move on to our last immune boosting tactic…

## Step 6 – Get More Sleep

Sleep is the best gift you can give your body. Most people are more susceptible to colds, the flu, viruses, bacterial infections and chronic fatigue when they don't sleep. There are many ways lack of sleep can interfere with your immune system. Let's look at some of them and come up with some common interventions that will help you get a better night of sleep.

### Trouble Sleeping

Many people have trouble falling or staying asleep. Often people have trouble falling asleep because:

➡ **They have too much on their mind**. To prevent going to sleep with a full head, start a journal you can review at night to help you release your worries before bed. You can't solve anything while sleeping, so put your worries to rest before you put yourself to bed.

- **They drink before bed.** Drinking before bed is a big mistake. Make sure you take your last (alcoholic) drink at least 4 hours before bed. Avoid caffeinated beverages up to 6 hours before you go to sleep. This will make a very noticeable difference in the way you sleep.

- **They exercise too close to bedtime.** You should exercise if you can first thing in the morning. Exercise in the morning gives your metabolism a boost for the day, and then allows you to sleep better at night. If you exercise too close to bedtime, you will feel too charged to sleep.

- **They watch television in bed.** The worst place to work or watch television is in bed. While it may "seem" comfortable, it can wreak havoc on your sleep. Some studies suggest the light from a television or the light emitted by a computer is enough to give a person chronic insomnia. This light tricks your brain into thinking it is time to wake up, so you have a harder time sleeping.

- **They eat too much protein before bed.** Protein is great for building muscle and boosting energy. If you want to sleep and stay asleep however, you might consider trying a low protein high carbohydrate snack sometime in the hour or two before bed. Make sure you do not eat too much because this too can interfere with sleep. A small snack however, may help keep your blood sugar levels aligned so you sleep better and longer. Many people find if they eat enough they do not wake nearly as often during the evening.

- **They suffer jet lag.** If you are a frequent flyer jet lag may be the cause of your insomnia. To help with this, ask your doctor about taking a melatonin supplement. This sometimes helps restore normal sleep patterns. You can also try adjusting your sleep schedule while on business or vacation so you do not mess up your normal sleep cycle rhythms. This may mean going to bed one or two hours earlier or later than normal, but most people would agree the change is worth it. Jet lag among frequent flyers is a concerning and almost disabling problem if not handled properly.

If you find you do not have enough time to sleep, then you have to work on your schedule to create more time to sleep. There is no such things as "catch up" sleep, so don't bother sleeping in extra on the weekends and working while sleep deprived during the week. It just doesn't work that way. You have to commit to a regular sleep routine to realize adequate results. If you do not have a sleep routine consider creating one.

Your goal is to get 7-8 hours of sleep ideally, although some people function well on 6-7 hours and others on 8-9 hours. Get to know your body, so you can determine how much sleep gets you where you need to be… feeling healthy and energetic during the day.

Sleep is a powerful tool. When we get enough sleep our bodies are better prepared to take on stress and disease. You will find you can conquer colds and infections much easier when you are fully rested. Make sure you sleep as much as you can especially when you are sick. You may find you need one or two extra hours of sleep when sick each day until better.

If this is true, get some sleep. Call in to work and tell them you are sick, whether you have sick time or not. Most managers and companies would prefer to have you working at optimum capacity rather than spreading disease throughout the company. Chances are high if you work while ill you will only increase the severity of your disease. You may then face a potentially serious infection, especially if you expose your weakened immune system to pollutants and bacteria on the job. Have you ever watched someone as they try to work while sick? Every sniffle and cough puts another person at risk for falling ill. Point that out to your manager if they give you trouble about staying home because of an illness.

Now you know some of the key tools for sleeping. Let's review some commonly asked questions so you get as much information as you need about health so you can boost your immune system and fight disease naturally.

## *Chapter 4 – Frequently Asked Questions*

Chances are high you still have some questions about your health and immune system. We will do our best to cover each of these in this section. If you still have questions that remain a puzzle, be sure to contact your healthcare provider so he or she can help you overcome whatever illness you struggle with.

This list contains some of the more commonly asked questions about immunity, sleep, stress and well-being.

**Q. Can I exercise while sick?**

**A.** Most people can engage in light exercise if they have a minor cold or feel only slightly ill. Be sure, however, if you do this to exercise very minimally. That means you can do with a walk around the park. You don't want to overdo it because this can cause you to feel sicker. You can sometimes help your body recover faster if you get a little exercise with a cold. If you are really sick however, and have a temperature above 99 degrees, you should call your doctor before trying to exercise. He or she will probably recommend you first rest and then try to exercise once you start feeling better.

**Q. I have a compromised immune system. What can I do to stay healthy?**

**A.** Many people suffer from compromised immune systems. Often the culprit is an autoimmune disease. This is a class of diseases where the body's immune system attacks healthy tissue instead of disease. This naturally causes fatigue. Certain medicines used to treat autoimmune disorders like lupus or rheumatoid arthritis may contribute to your susceptibility to illness. The best steps you can take are washing your hands frequently, encouraging others to do the same, using or carrying around a small bottle of sanitizer for your hands, and getting plenty of sleep so you can fight an infection if you happen to develop one.

If you have an autoimmune disorder, your doctor or rheumatologist may recommend you participate in continuous physical therapy which often can help your body recover and resist chronic illness. Be sure you cover your nose and mouth if needed when traveling to areas with large crowds or pollution. Having an autoimmune disorder is much like having an immature immune system (like a child has) or an immune system that is tired and overworked (as is sometimes the case with elderly patients).

Don't give up however. You can fight disease and feel better with time and good hygiene!

**Q. There are so many different recommendations for taking vitamin C. Some say you should take up to 4 grams each day. Won't this make you sick?**

**A.** Unfortunately there is much in the way of conflicting advice when it comes to caring for your body. The same is true of taking vitamin C. There are healthcare providers that swear you can take high doses of vitamin C to cure just about anything, from cold sores to cancer. Others suggest only a modest intake of vitamin C is worthwhile to the body.

Who do you listen to? You should always head the advice of your primary healthcare provider, someone you should trust, and your body. If you are taking too much vitamin C there is a good chance you will develop diarrhea. Your body usually takes as much vitamin C as it needs and expels the rest. Most people get plenty of vitamin C by eating fresh fruits and drinking fortified orange juice. When in doubt, less is probably best. Remember every body is different, so your body may react to vitamin C much quicker or slower than another person's body. Make sure you take time out to listen to your body.

**Q. Is Echinacea really helpful for boosting immunity? I heard it is just a
waste of time and money**.

**A**. Great question! The use of Echinacea is quite controversial. There are many
people that swear by its healing powers. There are studies that show it may help
shorten the duration of a cold or other virus. As with any study however, there
are an equal number that suggest Echinacea is no more beneficial than a
placebo. This is likely because different people respond differently to any
medication. Ask your doctor if you can try it. You usually need to take it at the
first hint of a cold. It does not help to take it daily, because it loses its
effectiveness after using it continuously for more than a month or so. Keep this in
mind.

**Q. Can I continue taking my supplements while ill?**

**A**. If your doctor prescribes medication for you regularly, or while you are ill, you
may need to stop your supplements until you finish your course of therapy. While
there are many herbs that safely combine with prescription and over-the-counter
medications, many do not. Ask a trained herbalist or medical doctor to help you
decide whether it is safe to take the medications you normally take with the
supplements or herbs you have. Remember, herbs are medicines too; they are
just natural medicines, the type that come from the ground. They should be
treated with the same care as you would any prescription medicine. If you notice
any side effects from an herb or supplement you take, be sure you report these
to your doctor immediately; you may have to switch medications or stop taking a
supplement.

# Conclusions

Congratulations! You are now on your way to healthy living. Taking care of your body is one of the best steps you can take to wellness and an excellent quality of life. Make sure you take care of your body as you would care for a child. You only get one chance to live in the skin you are currently in. There is no reason you need to damage your body to enjoy life.

Winter and spring are often the times when people become ill, usually resulting from viral infections or allergies. Make sure you get an annual or bi-annual check-up around these times so you can work with your doctor to prevent disease and illness, rather than just treat it. If you live a healthy lifestyle on a normal basis, the chances are high you will feel and look your best, day in and day out.

---

[i] Probiotic formula may bolster infant immune system, (2004). NUTRA, Europe. Available: http://www.nutraingredients.com/